THE FIFTYSOMETHING DIET

THE FIFTYSOMETHING DIET

How to Stay Healthy and Happy over Age 50

Next Avenue

ISBN-13: 978-1-62764-016-9
ISBN-10 1627640169

TABLE OF CONTENTS

INTRODUCTION

These days, there's no shortage of weight-loss programs or nutritional advice — media outlets are constantly releasing 'late-breaking' reports about dietary discoveries, many of which contradict previous recommendations. This makes it quite difficult for anyone to know what actions to take.

But if you are middle aged, there's an additional obstacle: Very little of what we read and hear is specifically geared to providing dietary and nutritional guidance for people age 50 and over. Yet, midlife is a time when natural physiological changes and the cumulative results of longstanding lifestyle habits demand that we rethink how we eat if we are to remain vital.

This eBook gathers advice and wisdom from blogs and articles written for nextavenue.org, a Web site designed for those in this new phase of life that we call Adult, Part 2. Next Avenue's Fiftysomething Diet takes direct aim at the nutritional needs of those in the second stage of adulthood. Each chapter presents dietary suggestions that can maximize physical and cognitive wellness in the face of the normal bodily shifts and increased risk of disease that occur with age.

Whether your goal is to shed pounds, boost energy, beat back dementia or generally maintain good health and a sense of well-being, The Fiftysomething Diet points the way.

THE FIFTYSOMETHING DIET

A health and aging specialist has developed a smart-eating system specifically for midlife

---

By Linda Dyett

Linda Dyett is a veteran writer and editor for magazines, newspapers and books who has written for a host of publications, including the New York Times, Psychology Today, Prevention , Oprah and Cosmopolitan.

Weight-loss programs and nutritional advice are more common today than ever before. But you'd be hard put to find an eating plan devised specifically for people age 50 and over — until now.

What may well lay claim as the world's first midlife diet is currently being deployed by George W. Yu, M.D., a surgeon and specialist in health and aging at Aegis Medical and Research Associates in Annapolis, Md., and the George Washington University Medical Center in Washington. By midlife, says Dr. Yu, "your body enters a different stage, and you must adjust your life and food choices to maintain your figure and your health."

To that end, Dr. Yu has developed a nutritionally sound tapas-and-global-fusion-food-oriented weight-reduction and maintenance regimen that is likely to appeal to the gastronomically savvy, who, like him, regard food as an adventure. It's got some iconoclastic surprises in it too, including exotic Eastern spices, small amounts of steak, even lightly buttered bread (once in a while) and the occasional binge meal.

This diet reflects Dr. Yu's hybrid cosmopolitan background: Born in Shanghai, raised in New York, trained in surgery at Harvard's Peter Bent Brigham Hospital, he worked in Cameroon, Kenya, Malawi and Honduras before going on to specialize in urological cancers at the Johns Hopkins Hospital in Baltimore.

It was witnessing the dramatic and dire effects of untimely hormone depletion in his cancer patients, men and women alike, that showed him how the loss of hormones like estrogen, progesterone and testosterone can lead to weight gain and the decay of bone and musculature (don't forget — the heart is a muscle). Hormone depletion occurs naturally, of course, during menopause and andropause, and plays a major role not only in women losing their hourglass figure and men their "V" shape, but also in sapping the vitality and strength of their earlier years.

But *disease enters through the mouth,* says Dr. Yu, quoting an ancient Chinese adage, and midlife digestibility plays an equally significant role in age-related weight gain, as well as muscle and bone loss. It's well known that starting in the 50s the stomach lining atrophies, and there is a slowdown in the production of stomach and pancreatic enzymes (which process nutrients) and in the movement of the intestinal tract.

This decline in digestibility makes you hungrier and puts you at risk for ill health downstream — from arthritis to cancers. "It's not a matter of bad genes," says Dr. Yu. "We've learned that genes don't express themselves unless conditions are right" — food, he says, being the most significant factor of all.

These aspects of the mechanics of aging are the bad news. The good news is that the effects of aging can be delayed, according to Dr. Yu. Specifically, he recommends daily exercises like cross-training, interval training and swimming. Swimming is especially beneficial, as lower underwater temperatures force the body to heat up and automatically burn off fat.

But the key, he says, is switching to a healthful diet. For his patients in midlife who are seeking both weight loss and optimal nutrition, Dr. Yu offers individualized eating regimens. These are some of his major tenets:

Restrict calories — but not the volume, texture, taste or nutritional value of the foods you eat. A proponent of the caloric-restriction regimen advanced by Roy Walford, the UCLA pathologist and Biosphere 2 crew member, Dr. Yu believes that cutting calories reduces the risk of disease and can extend life expectancy by as much as 30 percent. No surprise here, but what's out of the ordinary is his proposal of a cyclical diet. You start at 1,600 calories per day for two months. That's spartan, to be sure, but then you switch to two months at 2,200 calories per day.

"Being on a restricted calorie count alone will change your gene expression to a healthier state within four weeks," Dr. Yu maintains. And rotating these two calorie counts, he says, helps avoids the "nutritional boredom" that dooms many conventional diets

Go on a modified 24-hour fast every two months. This break from routine will give your intestinal tract — and your liver, especially — a rest. During the fast, it's okay to have a small serving of mild soup, rice porridge or mushy brown rice with a bit of flavoring. And drink plenty of water. Fasting produces a unique feeling of lightness and energy, says Dr. Yu.

Be a food rebel and diversify. Don't eat the same foods every day. Vary your meals and their ethnicity, so you're getting nutrients from a wide variety of vegetable and animal sources. The idea, says Dr. Yu, "is to mimic nature, but never let nature know what you're doing. Too much of the same thing produces resistance."

Drink at least a quart of water every day. Switch between mineral-rich tap water and nearly mineral-free reverse-osmosis water, such as Glaceau Smart Water. The body, Dr. Yu explains, needs ordinary water for optimal metabolism, while the reverse-osmosis variety reduces impurities. An ample water supply also decreases your risk of both constipation and headaches.

Have a substantial breakfast — your only big meal of the day — that's rich in protein and low in carbohydrates. To get protein, try a shake with whey, vegan or soy protein, as well as a poached egg — whose yolk isn't oxidized. For carbs, Dr. Yu recommends steel-cut oatmeal, buckwheat or short-grain brown rice with wild rice mixed in for texture. These grains may be cooked as porridge, but first they need to be soaked overnight — just as nuts and beans should be — to eliminate protease inhibitors (which block protein digestion) and phytates (mineral-blocking agents). Flavor with sesame powder, cinnamon or that antioxidant super-food, gogi berries.

Alternatively, have a serving of a not-too-sugary fruit, such as a Granny Smith apple or a mix of berries. Instead of coffee, which overstimulates the adrenal glands and weakens the stress hormones, drink herbal or green tea, or hot water with lemon or lime plus apple cider vinegar. Avoid fruit juice, which is much too sugary. If you crave the citrus flavor of orange juice, have an orange segment or two instead.

Eat six to seven small meals per day, each half the size of your fist. Freeing yourself of the lunch-and-dinner mindset will help you avoid sugar lows and insulin highs. Before you start eating a standard-size lunch, cut off half to save for a couple of hours later. Just doing this will automatically lower insulin and sugar levels. Yet you won't feel deprived, knowing the second half awaits you. Do the same split in the evening. If you're heading for a formal evening meal, have a snack two hours ahead, and eat just a small portion at the official dinner. After a month of half-and-half meals, Dr. Yu's patients often forget about the second helping.

Never get hungry. Snack on half a fistful or nuts and/or vegetable morsels (like cucumber slices). Some of Dr. Yu's patients have five small vegetable or nut snacks as an alternative to a big meal.

Nuts, in particular, are nutritionally dense, high in proteins and oils your body needs.

Have limited amounts of cholesterol. Cholesterol is the stuff that the sex hormones (still being produced after age 50, albeit in limited amounts), stress hormones, and vitamin D (technically a hormone — not a vitamin at all) are made of. It's part of every cell membrane in the body, and it insulates the nerves. For frying or spreading on the occasional slice of bread — or, preferably, a WASA whole-grain cracker — use judicious pats of butter. But don't overdo it.

Choose a variety of game and domestic meats — preferably from free-range animals — in paper-thin slices. To avoid eating meat in slabs, buy a kitchen scale and learn to downsize your portions. For most meals, aim for 3.5 ounces of meat, chicken, fish or seafood. Be sure to cut out any marbling fat (that's where toxic chemicals hide). One of Dr. Yu's favorites is paper-thin-sliced rare roast beef. Try it as a roulade, flavored with a sprinkling of sunflower or broccoli sprouts and a smidge of high-quality mustard or horseradish.

Eat bitter greens, as well as other vegetables. Bitter melon (the cucumber-shaped gourd with the bumpy surface, sold in Chinese markets), nopales (the insulin-lowering pads of the Mexican prickly pear), kale, brussels sprouts, broccoli, chard, collard greens, arugula, spinach, tatsoi (an Asian green with spoon-shaped leaves): All of the above clean out the liver and intestines and lower your sugar levels. Try them raw or quick-stirred, steamed, flavored with avocado, walnut, macadamia nut or coconut oil, Celtic sea salt, pepper or black bean sauce. Sunflower, broccoli and pea sprouts are the most nutritious greens with the fewest calories.

Switch to natural sweeteners like Stevia or brown-rice malt syrup. These sugar substitutes avoid the blood sugar surge, followed by an insulin surge.

To lower your sugar and insulin levels, take two gymnema tablets three times a day. Some professional literature indicates that gymnema (sold at health food stores) helps regenerate the pancreas's beta cells, which produce the insulin needed by the body to stave off sugar highs and diabetes.

Sprinkle anything sweet you eat with cinnamon. This spice also contains a chemical that lowers sugar and insulin levels.

Keep your wine consumption low. Wine may have health-giving benefits, but its sugar content is much too high, says Dr. Yu, who has treated many diabetic oenophiles.

Take a digestive enzyme supplement every day. This helps compensate for the loss of your own enzymes, and will minimize the bloating that often comes after a rich meal for those over age 50. Research has shown that these supplements shrink the pancreas's beta cells. Dr. Yu recommends the enzymes from Enzyme, Inc., available through medical and nutritional professionals.

MILK ALTERNATIVES — ARE THEY REALLY BETTER FOR YOU, OR IS IT HYPE?

What is really in almond, hemp seed, coconut, rice and soy milks

---

By Maureen Callahan

Maureen Callahan is a registered dietitian, recipe developer and lead author of the Health.com diet book review series.

Supermarket shelves are jammed with all manner of "milk" selections that don't come from the dairy down the road, but from plant sources like nuts, soy and grains. Rapidly stealing cows' milk customers, non-dairy beverages are popular for all kinds of reasons, from environmental concerns to animal well-being to lactose intolerance.

But what do these milk knock-offs taste like? And are they good-for-you? Looking at the big picture, it's a mix of pros and cons. On the plus side are low levels of artery-clogging saturated fat, zero cholesterol and convenient packaging. The cons: Sugar content is often high and protein levels, except in the case of soy milk, are not impressive. So before you start sipping, take a look at how some of these popular non-dairy beverages stack-up.

Almond Milk

The "Miss Congeniality" of non-dairy alternatives, almond milk glows with a nutrient-rich almond halo. After all, an ounce of almonds (23 nuts) sports a healthy six grams of protein, lots of Vitamin E and small amounts of minerals, like magnesium and calcium. The hitch: A cup of almond milk contains roughly four almonds, according to Nutrition Action Health Letter, barely enough to contribute much of that good-for-you almond nutrition. One cup of this milk (mostly water and sweeteners) delivers just one gram of protein, unless you buy one of the newer protein-fortified varieties. Bottom line: Drink it if you like the taste. (Note: All alternative milks have added sugars except for the unsweetened varieties.)

Calories per cup: 30-120; 1 gram protein, 1-23 grams carb (0-22 grams sugars), 3 grams fat

Sipping Notes: Lightly sweet with the faintest hint of almond.

Hemp Seed Milk

Fairly new to the non-dairy aisle, this light beige drink is winning over converts at a rapid clip, mostly due to its thicker, creamier texture. If you're a child of the '60s you might be connecting the dots and wondering if hemp has some of the same psychoactive compounds as marijuana. Not to worry. Hemp seeds contain zilch in the way of THC so they won't deliver that well-known "high." The nutrition claim to fame for these light-colored seeds is that they're a rich source of plant-based omega 3 fats, the kind of fats that are healthy for the heart. Of the 5-6 grams of fat in a cup of hemp milk, only half a gram is saturated fat. Alas, protein levels are low, just two grams per cup.

Calories per cup: 70-190; 2 grams protein, 1-35 grams carb (6-23 grams sugars), 6 grams fat

Sipping Notes: Mildly nutty with a subtle sweetness. Ranks as the thickest and creamiest of the milk alternatives, particularly the Tempt brand.

Coconut Milk

If you're expecting the big, bold flavor of canned coconut milk, this in-the-carton coconut beverage is sure to disappoint. It's hard to even detect coconut in the blend (unless you're one of those super tasters). What these drinks do have is plenty of saturated fat, ounce-for-ounce as much as whole milk. That probably explains their popularity as coffee creamers and cereal toppers since saturated fat delivers a richer mouthfeel. But is sipping saturated fat a good idea? Despite what you hear about coconut being a healthy fat, the American Heart Association still recommends going easy on all saturated fats, including coconut. Counting carbs? Coconut milk, which is low in protein like other alternatives, sports the lowest carb levels of alternative milks with a skimpy 5 or 6 grams of carbs on average. Even chocolate flavored varieties max out at 10 grams (a little over two teaspoons) of sugar.

Calories per cup: 50-100; 0-1 gram protein, 1-12 grams carb (1-10 grams sugars), 5 grams fat

Sipping Notes: Not very sweet and the coconut flavor is barely detectable.

Rice Milk

Made by blending cooked brown rice with water, this bright white drink looks most like cow's milk in the glass. But like other alternatives, it delivers a measly gram or two of protein per cup, compared to the 8 grams found in dairy milk. On the minus side for diabetics and anyone watching their sugar intake, it's also the richest in carbs of non-dairy beverages with unsweetened varieties often having 10 grams of carbs (instead of the usual one or two grams) and flavored varieties going as high as 34 grams (8 teaspoons sugar.) Who can benefit? Anyone with a nut allergy, or people looking for a gluten-free alternative.

Calories per cup: 70-160; 1-2 grams protein, 11-34 grams carb (1-28 grams sugars), 3 grams fat

Sipping Notes: Most "watery" of the alternative milks, this one is also the sweetest tasting.

Soy Milk

The best source of protein among the "milk" alternatives, soy milk is a close match to 2% cow's milk when it comes to nutrition. It carries about 7 grams of protein; cow's milk has 8 grams. It's moderate in fat, about 4 grams per cup, compared to 2% milk's 5 grams. Where they differ? Most of soy milk's fat is the unsaturated heart-healthy variety while most of cow's milk's fat is saturated. So if you're looking for a non-dairy beverage to replace milk's nutrition and improve on its fat profile, this is the one to buy. One caveat: Since most soybeans grown today are genetically modified, look for organic products if you want to sip "non-GMO."

Calories per cup: 90-130; 6-8 grams protein, 7-14 grams carb (6-11 grams sugar), 4 grams fat

Sipping Notes: Added sugars and flavors don't always do a good job of masking the mildly "beany" flavor.

Alternatives vs. Cow's Milk

Wondering about storage, safety, and cooking tips for your favorite alternative milk? Here are Next Avenue's answers to frequently asked questions:

How long do these milks last once opened?

Like cow's milk, most alternative milks are ultra pasteurized (exposed to high heat for short periods of time) to extend shelf life. Once opened, store them in the refrigerator and use them up in 7 to 10 days.

How can you tell if almond, rice or coconut "milk" is spoiled?

Just like with dairy products, alternative milks will curdle, develop funky aromas and go through changes in color and texture that signal spoilage.

Do these alternative milks match up to cow's milk when it comes to calcium and vitamin D?

That depends. Alternatives are fortified with anywhere from 10 to 45 percent of daily calcium requirements. But the type of calcium used is key. If it's calcium carbonate, the body takes it in easily. If it's tricalcium phosphate, don't expect to absorb as much due to lower bioavailability. Vitamin D is a slightly different story. Cow's milk is fortified with vitamin D3; alternatives contain vitamin D2, usually about 25 to 30 percent of the daily requirement. Which form of "D" is best? Both are well absorbed so either is a good source of the nutrient.

What's a good benchmark for healthy amounts of added sugar in these milks?

Unsweetened alternative milks, averaging 0 to 2 grams of sugar per cup, aren't a problem. And anything that keeps in line with cow's milk, which has 12 grams of natural sugars per cup, is probably fine. But step into flavored territory and sugar levels skyrocket. A cup of chocolate flavored almond or hemp seed milk packs a whopping 22 to 23 grams or almost 6 teaspoons of sugar. Chocolate-flavored rice milk can have as much as 34 grams of sugar. For reference, the American Heart Association recommends a daily limit of 6 teaspoons (24 grams) of added sugar calories per day for women and 9 teaspoons (36 grams) for men.

What's up with additives like guar gum, locust bean gum, tapioca starch and carrageenan?

Used in ice creams, puddings, and many packaged foods these generally recognized as safe (GRAS) chemicals are thickening agents used to improve mouthfeel and texture. Want to sidestep them and make your own alternative milks?

Can I bake and cook with non-dairy milks?

Yes and no. While most alternatives will stand in for dairy milk, results tend to be mixed. That makes sense when you consider that flavorings, sugar content, and thickeners — which vary from brand to brand and with each type of milk — can all impact the end result. Some general rules of thumb: Coconut milk and unsweetened milks work best in sauces. For baking, opt for milks with a similar sugar profile to cow's milk (12 grams of sugar per cup) since sugar impacts crust and texture. And check company websites for tips. Blue Diamond, for instance, advises against using Almond Breeze with packaged instant puddings.

Can I make yogurt with these milks?

Yes, although you might need extra thickeners to net a desirable yogurt texture.

5 FOODS YOU SHOULD NEVER EAT — OR TRY NOT TO!

Get these nutritional freeloaders out of your kitchen — they're not doing your body any good

---

By Maureen Callahan

Maureen Callahan is a registered dietitian, recipe developer and lead author of the Health.com diet book review series.

Suggesting that someone never eat certain foods tends to stir up a lot of angst. Surely the rare splurge on chocolate cake, French fries or any other tasty treat without nutritional merit isn't going to kill anybody, right?

Probably not. Yet, the reality is there are plenty of foods that aren't doing one bit of good for your fiftysomething body, pocketbook or even the planet. Simply put, they're just bad choices all around.

We've zeroed in on five of the biggest offenders, explaining why they're the perfect foods to pitch from your pantry and fridge, and to permanently cross off your shopping list.

1. Diet Soft Drinks

Ingredient Label for Diet Coke: *Carbonated water, caramel color, aspartame, phosphoric acid, potassium benzoate (preserves freshness), natural flavors, citric acid, caffeine.*

Over the last few years, researchers have linked diet soft drinks to everything from obesity to sugar cravings to depression. But a recent study in the Journal of General Internal Medicine suggests that routinely drinking these artificially sweetened soft drinks may do even more serious damage. They could increase your risk of vascular events like heart attack and stroke.

In the report, scientists followed for 10 years the soft-drink habits of more than 2,500 people over the age of 40. After accounting for other risk factors, like body mass index, high blood pressure and diabetes, researchers noticed that those who drank diet soft drinks on a daily basis were 43 percent more likely to suffer a vascular event, including heart attack and stroke, than people who drank none. The Harvard Health Letter does a nice job of summarizing the study and pointing out that more research is needed to confirm this link.

In the meantime, those in search of a flavorful replacement can sip on green teas, flavored and sparkling waters or iced coffee.

2. Luncheon Meats

Ingredient label for deli roast beef: *Beef, water, contains less than 2 percent of sodium lactate, slat, sodium phosphates, sodium diacetate, flavor, sodium ascorbate, sodium nitrite, caramel color.*

Slapping together a sandwich with a few slices of packaged, commercially processed deli meat on a daily basis can elevate your risk of developing colorectal cancer by 36 percent, according to a 2011 study from the American Institute for Cancer Research.

Scientists aren't certain if it's the nitrites, nitrates or other additives in these meats that confer the risk. They just point out that there is no amount of processed meat — including those preserved by smoking, salting or curing — that isn't associated with a higher incidence of cancer. The call to avoid this food category in its entirety dates to 2008, when the institute examined the findings from 7,000 studies and made its top 10 recommendations for preventing cancer.

"An occasional hot dog at a ball game, a festive ham at family gatherings — these aren't going to kill you," said Karen Collins, a nutritionist at the institute. "What we're cautioning against is making bacon, ham, sausage and lunch meat a part of your everyday pattern of eating. Enjoy these foods, but just limit them to a special occasion."

So what to put on a sandwich instead? The institute recommends leftover roasted chicken, grilled chicken breast, canned tuna or even hummus, combined with vegetables and fruits. Try sliced roast turkey breast, cranberry relish and sliced apples on toasted multigrain bread. Or a veggie wrap with hummus. Or tuna salad made with low-fat mayonnaise, celery and baby spinach leaves tucked into a whole-wheat pita.

3. Cool Whip

Ingredient Label for Cool Whip Regular: *Water, Hydrogenated Vegetable Oil (Coconut and Palm Kernel Oils), High Fructose Corn Syrup, Corn Syrup, Skim Milk, Light Cream, Contains less than 2 percent sodium caseinate, natural and artificial flavor, xanthan and guar gums, polysorbate 60, sorbitan monostearate, beta carotene (color).*

At some point, adding a dollop of real whipped cream to a cup of hot chocolate or a piece of pie became too much trouble for home cooks. In 1967, we were introduced to Cool Whip, a whipped-cream replacement that could keep in the refrigerator or be tossed in the freezer indefinitely. It took off like gangbusters, and now comes in five other versions, including extra creamy and sugar free. Late last year Cool Whip introduced Cool Whip Frosting to the product family. As convenient as these replacements may be, they're a mix of unhealthy hydrogenated oils, high fructose corn syrup and enough chemical additives to make you squirm.

In a Cool Whip experiment, a New York dad left the topping out on the counter at room temperature for 12 days and found that it looked exactly the same as day one in the refrigerator. Of course, this isn't strong science, but it does make you wonder how the body feels about this foreign concoction.

Better to get out the bowl and beaters. One tablespoon of real whipped cream sports just 26 calories and 1.7 grams of saturated fat. (If you like it sweet, a tiny amount of sugar will do the trick for a large quantity). By comparison, one tablespoon of Cool Whip has 25 calories and 1.5 grams of saturated fat. In other words, they're almost identical. But the occasional splurge on real whipped cream is a natural alternative that tastes a whole lot better.

4. Cooking Spray

Ingredient Label for Pam Cooking Spray: *Organic Canola Oil (Adds a Trivial Amount of Fat), Organic Grain Alcohol (Added for Clarity), Lecithin from Soybeans (Prevents Sticking), Propellant (No Chlorofluorocarbons).*

While the Food and Drug Administration says the propellant gases used in cooking oil sprays are safe food additives, we take issue with how much fat these sprays really save you, along with the cost to your wallet and cookware. A 2012 review from Cook's Illustrated finds that putting your own oil in a mister costs about 9 cents per ounce, compared with 60 cents per ounce for a cooking spray like Pam. (Or you can purchase a top-of-the-line canola oil — cold-pressed, organic, GMO free — from Amazon.com that's a mere 20 cents per ounce.)

Then there's that icky brown residue sprays can leave on muffin tins, cookie sheets and nonstick pans when temperatures get a little too hot. It's a polymer residue that can't be removed.

But assuming these sprays are low fat is probably the biggest mistake. The consumer watchdog group Center for Science in the Public Interest says "a ridiculously tiny serving size of a third, a quarter, or even a fifth of a second spray helps Pam and other aerosol cooking sprays boast zero calories and zero fat, even though the products are mostly fat." A more realistic six-second spray adds up to 6 grams of fat and 50 calories. For comparison, one teaspoon of canola oil has 40 calories and 4.5 grams of fat.

Bottom line: What's so hard about drizzling a teaspoon of real oil — minus additives and propellant — into a nonstick skillet, or wiping some oil into muffin tins with your fingers? Think olive, canola, coconut and sesame oil — and peanut oil, which doesn't depart flavor when heated.

5. Steam-in-the-Bag Vegetables

Ingredients for steam-in-the-bag peas: peas.

Water bottles, plastic cups and cans lined with hard plastics made with a chemical called Bisphenol A, or BPA, came under fire a few years ago. Animal studies showed exposure to these compounds, which can leach into food when heated, might create multiple health problems, including reproductive disorders, diabetes and cardiovascular disease.

The government is still unsure of the risks associated with BPA. But those animal studies are making many people wonder about the safety of all kinds of plastics that come into contact with hot food. "When food is wrapped in plastic or placed in a plastic container and microwaved, substances used in manufacturing the plastic (plasticizers) may leak into the food. In particular, fatty foods such as meats and cheeses cause a chemical called diethylhexyl adipate to leach out of the plastic," says the Harvard Health Letter.

The amount of leakage, the article points out, is small; the FDA, which monitors containers for safety, allows for this small migration of plasticizer compounds. But who knows what these small doses will do to you — so why risk it? It takes no time to transfer frozen vegetables into a glass container before microwaving them.

5 FOODS THAT WILL BRING YOUR BLOOD PRESSURE DOWN

Consuming natural foods, along with cutting out salt, will have you eating well and avoiding heart disease

---

By Janet Bond Brill, Ph.D

Janet Bond Brill, Ph.D., is the author of 'Blood Pressure Down: The 10-Step Plan to Lower Your Blood Pressure in 4 Weeks Without Prescription Drugs' (Three Rivers, 2013). A registered dietitian, she is also spokeswoman for the American Heart Association's Go Red for Women movement.

High blood pressure, also known as "the silent killer," is an epidemic in our nation. It typically has no warning signs or symptoms, and many people don't realize they have it, which is why we must all get it checked regularly. Over time, unaddressed elevated blood pressure can have disastrous consequences including stroke, heart attack, blindness and kidney failure.

Every 39 seconds, someone in this country dies of cardiovascular disease. And despite the fact that the largest risk factor in these deaths — high blood pressure — is both preventable and reversible, as many as 67 million American adults live with high blood pressure, according to the federal Centers for Disease Control and Prevention. Alarmingly, 47 percent of those with a diagnosis have not gotten their blood pressure under control, according to government research. And many of those afflicted don't adhere to recommended medication regimens because of the drugs' side effects.

Medications are highly effective in bringing down blood pressure, when taken properly. But what you eat (and drink) also has a dramatic impact. The government-endorsed Dietary Approaches to Stop Hypertension (DASH) diet has been proven as effective as prescription medication in reducing blood pressure.

Many imagine that a blood-pressure-lowering diet involves bland, unseasoned foods and deprivation. That couldn't be further from the truth. Although reducing your sodium intake is an important step in lowering blood pressure, what you add to your diet is as important as what you take out.

Here are 5 surprising and delicious foods from my Blood Pressure DOWN action plan:

Bananas The most popular fruit in the United States, bananas are delectable, portable, inexpensive and filled with fiber. Each banana also has at least 450 milligrams of potassium, nature's most powerful blood-pressure-lowering medicine.

To bring your blood pressure down, you need to go beyond slashing salt and ingest more potassium as well. Abundant scientific evidence has proven that a shortage of this electrolyte plays a major role in the onset of high blood pressure and that restricting potassium intake can cause a blood pressure spike even among people with no previous concerns. A low potassium intake also ups your odds of suffering a stroke.

In practice, potassium offsets the harmful effects of sodium. To lower your blood pressure through dietary means, you need to shift your body's balance of sodium and potassium by bringing your sodium intake to under 1500 milligrams a day while raising your potassium intake to about 4700 milligrams — the average American adult consumes only about half this much today. (Diabetics, people with chronic kidney disease and those taking a blood thinner, like warfarin, should check with their doctor before increasing their potassium intake.) Potassium is also a natural diuretic — so the more you eat, the more sodium and water you'll excrete through urine.

Avocado Another potassium powerhouse, the avocado, contains 975 milligrams of the mineral. It also delivers a variety of other heart-healthy vitamins, minerals, phytonutrients and monounsaturated fat. Try a ripe avocado on a sandwich instead of mayonnaise or butter and you'll be doing your heart a service by replacing artery-clogging fats with a super-buttery, creamy and tasty spread. Or try a simple guacamole recipe — packed with blood-pressure-lowering nutrients. Serve it as a dip with low-salt bagel or pita chips, or as an accompaniment to quesadillas or tacos.

Yogurt The science is in: Adults who consume 1000 to 1500 milligrams of calcium a day in their food reduce their risk of contracting high blood pressure, according to studies of the DASH diet. (Most of us come up woefully short of that target now.) So what's better — taking a supplement or eating calcium-rich foods? One comprehensive meta-analysis by the Women's Health Initiative found that a tailored high-calcium diet had twice the blood-pressure-lowering effect of a calcium-supplement regimen. (Post-menopausal women should still discuss supplements with their doctor to reduce their risk of bone fractures.)

How can you possibly get enough calcium from food? Start with the richest source out there — plain nonfat yogurt — and eat two or more cups a day. Yogurt can also keep your digestive system in tune by supplying live, "friendly" probiotic bacteria, like Lactobacillus acidophilus and Bifidobacterium lactis, which promote intestinal function. You can also try yogurt in vegetable or fruit dips, atop your morning bowl of oatmeal or in place of water in pancake and other baked-good recipes. You'll be surprised how this simple swap adds both taste and nutrition.

Dark Chocolate What gives dark chocolate its blood-vessel benefits? Polyphenols, a major class of bioactive phytochemicals proven to protect against heart and vascular disease. Flavonoids, a subclass of polyphenols that accounts for about two-thirds of our polyphenol intake, are found in high concentration in dark chocolate, as well as in fruits and vegetables. To satisfy your chocolate craving and lower your blood pressure, go with the real thing.

Natural unsweetened cocoa powder has the highest concentration of flavonoids of any chocolate product, followed by unsweetened baking chocolate. Cocoa powder is also lower in sugar, fat and calories than solid chocolate bars.

Red Wine Too much alcohol increases your risk of high blood pressure and a host of other health concerns. But in moderation (and only in moderation), red wine soothes the arteries, reduces blood sugar and lessens your diabetes risk. The Department of Agriculture defines moderate consumption of wine as one five-ounce glass per day for women and up to two per day for men. This small amount of red wine daily, with food, is part of an evolving lifestyle prescription for preventing the onset of high blood pressure and even addressing existing hypertension.

The key is the presence of substances believed to lower blood pressure in combination — ethyl alcohol (ethanol) and antioxidant polyphenols, including resveratrol and procyandins. To get the most out of wine's cache of polyphenols, though, stick with red varieties, which average 10 times the polyphenol content of whites because they are fermented with the skins and seeds of the grape.

One additional advantage of enjoying a glass of wine with dinner: It encourages you to slow down, relax and truly savor your meal.

5 POWERFUL WEIGHT-LOSS BOOSTERS

Science is finding that these foods and drinks can help you shed pounds more easily and quickly

---

By Maureen Callahan

Maureen Callahan is a registered dietitian, recipe developer and lead author of the Health.com diet book review series.

Staying at a healthy weight during your fiftysomething years is a balancing act between calories consumed and burned. Chances are you already know that you need fewer calories as you age. So it's trickier to prevent weight gain without making some efforts. Exercise is one good strategy, especially aerobic activities, like brisk walking, swimming, dancing and biking. But it also pays to take advantage of any and all foods that can burn fat, curb appetite and tweak your metabolism into overdrive. Here's a look at five foods that do just that.

1. **Dried Beans** Foods rich in water-soluble fiber, like kidney beans, chickpeas and black beans, not only help you feel full at meals but they may even target your stubborn spare tire. In a 2011 study, researchers noticed that for every 10 grams of soluble fiber eaten over the course of a day there was a corresponding 3.7 percent decrease in abdominal fat over a five-year period.

"There is mounting evidence that eating more soluble fiber and increasing exercise reduces visceral or belly fat, although we still don't know how it works," said Dr. Kristen Hairston, assistant professor of internal medicine at Wake Forest Baptist Medical Center in North Carolina and lead author of the study. "Although the fiber-obesity relationship has been extensively studied, the relationship between fiber and specific fat deposits has not. Our study is valuable because it provides specific information on how dietary fiber, especially soluble fiber, may affect weight accumulation through abdominal fat deposits."

2. **Salmon** One of the biggest food helpers on the path to weight loss is protein — preferably lean protein, which is better for the heart and overall health. The simple explanation is that a good dose takes longer to digest than carbohydrates, keeping you satisfied and therefore making you less likely to overeat between meals. It doesn't hurt that the body burns more calories digesting proteins than it does carbs. But the intriguing thing about fish as your protein source — salmon, in particular — is that preliminary reports suggest salmon plays a role in modulating insulin levels or insulin sensitivity.

The key word here is preliminary. Still, two reports bear mentioning. In one 2009 study, scientists fed three groups of volunteers low-calorie diets: no seafood (the control group), lean white fish or salmon. Everyone lost weight, but the salmon eaters had lower fasting insulin levels, which is far better for overall health. Weight loss is one partial explanation, researchers say, but the compounds in salmon (perhaps omega 3 fats like EPA and DHA) might also contribute to modulating insulin.

In an unrelated 2011 study with animals, Canadian researchers found that a group fed salmon protein had significantly lower weight gains than groups eating other varieties of fish. What's happening here is still part mystery, yet it could be a win-win. Choosing salmon as your lean protein source might not only help you lose weight, but also help prevent the insulin resistance that can lead to type 2 diabetes in later years.

Wild salmon is leaner than farmed. It contains plenty of protein minus unhealthy fats. Three ounces of cooked wild salmon contains 155 calories, 22 grams of protein and just 7 grams of fat, most of it the heart-healthy omega 3 variety.

3. Nuts Most dieters shy away from nuts due to their high fat content, but research suggests almonds, peanuts and other nuts offer special weight loss benefits. It all started with a 2001 landmark study from Harvard that found that participants following a Mediterranean-style diet that included nuts and peanuts lost greater amounts of weight and stuck with the diet longer than those on a different low-fat diet. (Harvard researchers now call the Mediterranean plan the best way to lose weight and keep it off.)

Then a 2003 study in the International Journal of Obesity discovered that an almond-eating group of overweight volunteers (eating 85 grams per day or about 3 ounces) lost 62 percent more weight and 56 percent more body fat than a nut-free diet group eating the exact same number of calories but no nuts. Research also confirms that women who eat nuts have lower body mass indexes, or BMI, than women who eat little or no nuts. Speculation is that the fat and protein in nuts helps keep dieters full longer.

Whatever the reason, all researchers say the key watchword is moderation — say, a couple of small handfuls of nuts a day. Count on a handful being about one ounce of nuts: 157 pine nuts, 49 pistachios, 24 almonds, 20 walnut halves, 20 pecans, 20 hazelnuts, 18 cashews or 12 macadamia nuts. Keep in mind, you can nullify all health benefits if nuts are covered with chocolate, sugar or salt.

4. Green Tea We've mentioned before that green tea contains antioxidants (called polyphenols) that may fight cancer and lower cholesterol levels. But studies suggest it might be time to add fat burner — or maybe we should say belly buster — to the list of health benefits.

Scientists seem to be zeroing in on a specific group of polyphenol compounds called catechins as the surprising force behind weight loss. A 2009 study from the Journal of Nutrition showed that a group of 132 overweight and obese adults doing moderate exercise for 180 minutes per week and drinking either a caffeinated beverage with green tea catechins or a control beverage with no catechins, had remarkably different weight-loss scenarios. At the end of 12 weeks, the exercisers drinking green tea with 625 milligrams of catechins lost more weight and more belly fat and had lower triglyceride levels than dieters drinking the catechin-free beverage.

It's unclear how green tea promotes weight loss, but researchers suspect it may have something to do with revving up fat burning in the hours after a meal. A small 2013 Brazilian study confirms these findings. Researchers there found that overweight and obese women drinking green tea and following a program of resistance training lost more body fat, lowered their waist circumference and showed more significant increases in their resting metabolic rate than women who drank a placebo or green tea but didn't exercise.

Bottom line: To net the fat-burning efforts of green tea it appears you need to pair your tea sipping with exercise.

5. Water Call it the forgotten weight loss aid, but studies continue to confirm that good old zero-calorie H2O is one of the cheapest and most effective weight-loss aids on the planet.

Will it work on a fiftysomething body? Definitely.

A 12-week 2010 Virginia Tech Study divided a group of overweight adults age 55-75 into two groups. All participants ate the same amount of calories, but half the group was asked to drink two cups of water before each meal; the other half drank no water. "We found that over the course of 12 weeks, dieters who drank water before meals, three times per day, lost about 5 pounds more than dieters who did not increase their water intake," said Brenda Davy, an associate professor in the College of Agriculture and Life Sciences at Virginia Tech, senior author on the study.

Davy says the exact mechanism responsible for weight loss is uncertain. She speculates it could be as simple as the fact that water fills up the stomach and makes you feel like eating less. In an earlier study, she and colleagues noticed that middle-aged and older adults who drank two cups of water before a meal ended up eating about 75-90 fewer calories. Another plus of choosing water as your beverage of choice before meals: There's less room for calorie-rich options like soda, sugary cocktails or fruit juice.

5 SEEDS YOU NEED TO EAT

Discover the super health benefits of flavorful, nutrient-rich kernels, including those found in sunflowers, flax and hemp

By Maureen Callahan

Maureen Callahan is a registered dietitian, recipe developer and lead author of the Health.com diet book review series.

When it comes to smart foods in small packages, nuts like almonds and walnuts tend to hog the spotlight. But there's a whole other arsenal of other tasty, nutrient-dense foods you might want to tap into — seeds. They may be tiny but they're nutritional powerhouses loaded with healthy fats, fiber, protein and minerals. Supercharge your diet by snacking on these five seeds and sprinkling them into your dishes.

1. **Chia** Forget about "ch-ch-ch-chia pet plants." The ancient Aztec chia is making a strong comeback as a "hip" food ingredient. Eat the seeds raw on their own or add to almost any kind of food, like juice, yogurt, soup, eggs, pancakes, salad dressing and smoothies.

Nutrients A whopping 10 grams of fiber in one tablespoon is a good start. But chia seeds pack a whole lot more in their little round package. So count on good amounts of protein, iron, calcium, magnesium, zinc and plenty of those plant-based omega-3 fats (alpha linolenic acids).

The Newest Research Despite the hype, a 2012 study suggests that eating chia seeds isn't a "cure" for what ails you, at least in the short term. "It didn't magically change disease risk factors," Appalachian State University researcher David Nieman said in a North Carolina paper. "It isn't like taking a pill to lower your cholesterol." Nor does it help with weight loss, as Nieman and colleagues found in an earlier 2009 study. It's just a good, nutrient-rich food.

A Few Tips

- Soaking chia seeds in fruit juice or water allows them to swell to several times their initial size and become gelatinous, a plus for people who want their beverages, puddings and cereals to be more filling.
- New research suggests seeds need to be milled to release plant-based omega-3 fats. That's because your body may not get the benefits of the whole seeds if your digestive track can't break them down. Milling them — aka grinding them into a flour — is needed to "release" the good nutrition.

2. **Flax** Food companies may add them whole to snacks, but the only way to open yourself up to the health benefits of these tiny, nutty-flavored seeds is to grind them (or buy them already ground into flaxseed meal). Try them in a healthy smoothie or sprinkled on yogurt and cereal. And don't worry about seed color. Dark brown or golden-hued, the nutrition profile is identical.

Nutrients Rich in plant-based omega-3 fats, each 35-calorie tablespoon of ground flaxseed meets government guidelines for alpha linolenic acid — 1.1 grams per day for women and 1.6 grams per day for men. Also, count on that same tablespoon giving you 1 to 2 grams of soluble fiber, a big reason why flax is considered such a good laxative.

The Newest Research A 2012 study by the American Heart Association finds that eating an ounce of ground flaxseed daily for six months can lower blood pressure. Some small studies find the seed might help protect against prostate cancer and a 2013 Canadian study reports a link between eating flaxseed and reduced breast cancer risk.

A Few Tips

- Flaxseed can stand in for eggs in pancakes or baked goods; mix 2 tablespoons of ground flaxseed with 3 tablespoons of water to replace each egg.
- There have been some reports of drug-flaxseed interactions so check with your doctor if you take statins, blood thinners, NSAIDs or the antibiotic cyclosporin.

3. **Sunflower Seeds** The beautiful yellow flower is a sight to behold, but its real gold can be found in its black-and-white hulled seeds. Great for snacking or as a topping for cereal, crisps and yogurt. Or chop them into a healthy coating for pan-fried chicken tenders.

Nutrients An ounce (1/4 cup) of shelled seeds delivers one-third of the daily requirement for vitamin E and phosphorous. That same 170-calorie serving also offers up small amounts of protein, fiber, zinc, folate, vitamin B6 and choline, which has been linked to better memory and cognitive performance in older adults.

The Newest Research A large 2012 German study notes a reduced risk of breast cancer among postmenopausal women who eat high amounts of sunflower seeds, pumpkin seeds and soybeans, compared to women who don't eat those foods.

A Few Tips

- Consider avoiding sunflower seeds if you have a latex allergy since they could put you at increased risk for an IgE-mediated, food-induced reaction.

- Resist stirring seeds into muffin or quick bread batters made with baking soda — the two ingredients chemically interact to tint baked goods a harmless, but unappealing, blue-green hue.

4. Pumpkin Seeds (Pepitas) Raw pumpkin seeds are a rich, green color, but they turn brown when toasted. Easily found in whole food or natural grocery stores, they make a crunchy topping for baked goods, yogurt and cereals.

Nutrients An ounce of roasted pumpkin seeds has 126 calories, 5 grams of protein and 5.5 grams of fat, giving it the skinniest nutrition profile of the seed family. Like other seeds, they're also a good source of minerals, including magnesium, potassium and zinc.

The Newest Research As mentioned above, a recent German study reported a reduced risk of breast cancer among postmenopausal women who eat high amounts of pumpkin seeds, sunflower seeds and soybeans. In a 2011 study, Jamaican researchers noticed higher levels of HDL, or "good" cholesterol, and improvement in menopausal symptoms for women supplementing their diets with pumpkin seed oil.

A Few Tips

- For a healthy snack, buy raw pepitas and toast them with lime juice and a spice rub.
- Or save seeds from a pumpkin and roast them yourself.

5. Hemp Seeds At $15 a pound or more, tiny hemp seeds are pricey little devils. But their high-quality protein and stellar nutrition numbers make them a heavenly choice for anyone following a plant-based diet.

Nutrients The big plus of hemp seeds, a factor that separates them from all others, is that they're a complete protein, one of the few plant foods that contain all nine essential amino acids or building blocks of protein. Also noteworthy: generous amounts of vitamin E, plant-based omega-3 fats and minerals, including phosphorus, potassium, sodium, magnesium, sulfur, calcium, iron and zinc. Two tablespoons contain 90 calories, 6 grams of fat, 5 grams of protein and 2 grams of fiber.

The Newest Research Just about everything in their nutrition profile suggests hemp seeds might help protect against heart disease and other ills. But we don't have a lot of research to support what hemp seeds can do. That's because people and food companies have shied away from a food plant that is related to marijuana. When in reality there are no marijuana-like effects to be had from hemp seeds. They are entirely safe.

A Few Tips

- New to most kitchens, look for recipes using hemp seeds at Vegetarian Times
- Or try this Fruit and Hemp Seed Muesli.

5 NUTRIENTS YOU NEED RIGHT NOW

Fortify your diet with vitamins D and B12, omega-3 fatty acids and two essential minerals

By Debra Witt

Debra Witt is a lifestyle writer and editor with a background covering the latest news, trends, and personalities in health, fitness, fashion, and beauty.

In a recent article, 5 Myths About Nutritional Supplements, we shot down the myth that you need to be taking multiple single-nutrient supplements every day. But we also pointed out that, depending on your overall health and diet, there are some possible exceptions.

The experts we consulted identified five nutrients that many of us may not be getting in sufficient amounts through our meals alone. All are crucial to our health. Some can be obtained through supplements. Others we can get through our diet, although we may need to make adjustments.

1. Calcium

Recommended Daily Value: 1,000 mg for men over 50; 1,200 mg for women over 50 and everyone over 70. (As you get older, you need more because your ability to absorb the nutrient from food gradually declines.)

Why you need it: Your body needs calcium to maintain bone mass, and it helps your muscles expand and contract. Calcium also helps regulate the pH level of your blood, aids in the production of many hormones and enzymes, and contributes to healthy blood pressure.

How to get it: Three daily servings of dairy (such as milk, yogurt, cheese), plus one serving of another calcium-rich food, like fortified cereal, sardines, salmon, fortified orange juice or a soy beverage. Dietitian Joan Salge Blake, a professor at Boston University and a spokesperson for the Academy of Nutrition and Dietetics, says most of us should be able to get our daily needs through our food: One cup of nonfat milk, sipped with a meal, provides almost 900 mg, for example. Add a two-ounce serving of cheese and you've met the RDV. Another option: a calcium supplement. It's best to get your calcium throughout the day, though, so even if you take it as a supplement, divide it into two doses a day, with meals.

2. Vitamin D

Recommended Daily Value: 600 IU (international units) for adults up to age 70; 800 IU for adults over 71.

Why you need it: The body needs vitamin D to absorb calcium. It also helps to transport messages between the brain and the rest of the body — with vitamin D receptors in just about every cell in the body, taking in optimal amounts helps maintain the body's communication system. But your skin, liver and kidney's ability to produce vitamin D declines with age, and low levels of the nutrient affect our hunger signals, mood, immune system and more.

How to get it: The best way to generate vitamin D is through exposure to the sun, which aids production of the nutrient in your body. But UV rays are strong enough to boost vitamin D production only between 10 a.m. and 3 p.m. — prime working hours for many adults. What's more, the sun needs to hit more than your hands and face, and even when we're not covered up, most of us wear sunscreen, which is the right choice — it just means we need to get our vitamin D in other ways. Most milk today is fortified with D (about 400 IU per quart), as are many brands of orange juice, yogurt and cereal (amounts vary).

Vitamin D is also found in fatty fish, but you'd need to incorporate it into two meals in order to hit the daily goal. With relatively limited natural sources, then, many of us rely on vitamin D supplements. Nutrition and health experts have been debating the proper daily dose, based on emerging studies that show a possible link between the nutrient and benefits such as a stronger immune system, reduced inflammation and fracture prevention. Some now recommend a daily 1,000 IU dose; others resist raising their recommendation because of a small but measurable risk of developing kidney stones.

3. Magnesium

Recommended Daily Value: 420 mg for men over 30; 320 mg for women over 30.

Why you need it: The mineral is necessary for a healthy immune system, to maintain bone and muscle mass and nerve function, to regulate your heart rate and more. Yet three out of four adults over the age of 50 don't get enough, says dietitian Elizabeth Somer, author of *Eat Your Way to Sexy* (Harlequin, 2011).

How to get it: Magnesium is abundant in wheat germ, whole grains, nuts and leafy greens. Women would need to eat two cups of cooked spinach or four ounces of almonds or cashews to reach that target. If that's more than you're willing to consume, Somer recommends getting the mineral from a multivitamin (check for magnesium on the label) or a calcium supplement that is two parts calcium, one part magnesium.

4. Vitamin B12

Recommended Daily Value: 2.4 micrograms (mcg).

Why you need it: Vitamin B12 helps produce DNA and protects our nerve and blood cells. But as we age, our stomachs secrete less of the hydrochloric acid that's necessary to absorb B12 from our food, Salge Blake says. We can absorb the B12 that comes from supplements and fortified foods, though.

How to get it: B12 is found naturally in animal foods, especially beef liver and clams, and in some fortified foods. We can also get it from a multivitamin that contains about 100 percent of the RDV of B12.

5. Omega-3 Fatty Acids (fish oil)

Recommended Daily Value: 220 mg DHA (docosahexaenoic acid).

Why you need it: The omega-3 fatty acid DHA is essential for brain function and also plays a key role in reducing your risk of heart disease. One recent large-scale study, known as the MIDAS study, found that older people who got 900 mg of DHA daily showed improved memory function after six months, compared with those who took a placebo.

How to get it: Eating two eight-ounce portions a week of fatty fish (salmon, mackerel, sardines) is the best way to meet your needs, Salge Blake says. One whole serving of cooked salmon, for example, provides 1.2 grams of DHA. If you're not a regular fish eater and you're considering an omega-3 supplement, Salge Blake advises that you consult your doctor or a registered dietitian for guidance on the proper dose (or, for that matter, about starting to take any dietary supplement).

Your doctor may recommend you take a supplement just a couple of times a week, as it's easy to consume too much DHA and high doses can cause gastric distress, or interfere with medications.

For example, DHA may interfere with blood clotting in people who take a daily aspirin or blood thinner.

Get Advice From the Right Sources

There seem to be news reports every day about new dietary discoveries and breathless recommendations. Some should lead to changes in your diet; the benefits of others may still be unproven. To find out what you actually need to do, consult your doctor, or a registered dietitian. Many health insurance plans cover dietitian visits. Depending on your plan, simply being over 50 may qualify you for one or more covered sessions. If you're being treated for high blood pressure, high cholesterol, diabetes or other chronic conditions, the likelihood that your insurance will cover a consultation is even higher. To find a dietitian near you, go to eatright.org and click "Find a Registered Dietitian."

10 YUMMY, HEALTHY SNACKS

You can munch these healthful snacks to your heart's content (and your waistline's!)

By Maureen Callahan

Maureen Callahan is a registered dietitian, recipe developer and lead author of the Health.com diet book review series.

Everyone loves to snack, but we all know what the wrong between-meal nosh can do to you, especially after the age of 50. Too much salt and your blood sugar zooms out of control. Too high a dose of saturated fat and your arteries clog up. Just a few too many calories — even, say, a small bowl of ice cream with the tiniest spoonful of hot fudge sauce — and before you know it your calorie-conserving fiftysomething body starts putting on the pounds. It's just not fair.

But you don't have to give up snacking. The trick is to become a little pickier. Search out tasty nibbles that don't go overboard on calories and that are chock-full of vitamins, minerals, fiber and anti-oxidants — ingredients that can help keep the mind sharp, muscles strong and energy levels high. Topping that list: fresh fruits, veggies, whole grains, "good" fats and lean proteins. In other words, you may not be able to have your Doritos and eat them too, but there are plenty of healthful options that your body will thank you for.

By mixing and match beneficial ingredients, snacks don't have to be one-note or boring.

Here are 10 snacks that will not only satisfy the health needs of your fiftysomething body, they'll also taste better than many store-bought, high-fat, overly processed alternatives.

1. Peanut Butter-Banana Crisp (180 calories)

Crunchy whole-grain crackers are a wholesome snack when topped with a tablespoon of nut butter and half a sliced banana. The best whole-grain crackers? Any that are fiber-rich and low in calories, including Wasa and Ryvita crispbread. Need gluten-free? Mary's Gone Crackers or Brown Rice Crackers are good options.

The healthy bottom line: A balanced mix of protein, fiber and heart-healthy unsaturated fats, plus a good dose of blood pressure-lowering potassium from the banana.

2. Sugar Snap Peas & Cherry Tomatoes With Hummus (157 calories)

Carrot sticks are great dippers. But go one step better and broaden the color spectrum with other raw or lightly steamed vegetables. Fresh sugar snap peas (you can get them pre-washed), bell pepper strips, asparagus — it's all good. Aim for about a cup of veggies and 1/4 cup of any flavored hummus.

The healthy bottom line: All kinds of nutrients, fiber and disease-fighting compounds in the veggies, and a little protein and good fat in the hummus.

3. Cottage Cheese & Blueberries (163 calories)

Salty cottage cheese (a good source of protein) makes a perfect backdrop for sweet, fresh berries. Dish out one-half cup of 1 percent reduced-fat cottage cheese and cover it with one cup of blueberries, raspberries, strawberries or blackberries.

The healthy bottom line: New studies find eating antioxidant-rich berries can put the skids on cognitive decline and lower the risk of developing Parkinson's disease.

4. Greek Yogurt, Fruit & Nuts (169 calories)
Is your sweet tooth calling? Start with creamy, zero-fat plain Greek-style yogurt and sweeten it naturally by stirring in one chopped kiwi and a few blackberries (1/4 cup). Top with 1 tablespoon of toasted sliced almonds. Not sweet enough? Drizzle with a teaspoon (20 calories) of honey, maple syrup or agave nectar.

The healthy bottom line: The plain, zero-fat Greek yogurt has twice the protein and none of the blood-sugar-raising additives of sweetened yogurts. The kiwi delivers a day's worth of immune-strengthening vitamin C. And the almonds are rich in vitamin E.

5. Apple & Cashew Butter (176 calories)
Slice one medium apple and serve with 1 tablespoon of any nut butter — peanut, sunflower seed, cashew — for dipping. It's a perfect snack for the office or backpack since there's no refrigeration required.

The healthy bottom line: The apple has cholesterol-lowering soluble fiber and a dozen different nutrients. Nut butter delivers protein and heart-healthy fat.

6. Raisin, Cranberry & Peanut Gorp (183 calories)
Tuck away 2 tablespoons of raisins, 1 tablespoon of dried, sweetened cranberries and 2 tablespoons of roasted, salted peanuts into mini plastic snack bags for on-the-go munching. (Yes, salted nuts are okay here, since amounts are small. Two tablespoons of oil-roasted, salted peanuts deliver 78 milligrams of sodium, about half as much as a slice of bread.)

The healthy bottom line: Cardiologists say raisins (rich in potassium, fiber, phenols, tannins and antioxidants) can help lower blood pressure. Pair them with heart-healthy peanuts for double the positive punch.

7. Edamame (150 calories)
Served in the pod (like peanuts), edamame — or boiled green soybeans — have a slightly nutty, sweet flavor. Find them in the supermarket freezer section and fill up on 3/4 cup of shelled beans (or 1.5 cups of unshelled pods) for one of the best all-around, fill-you-up snacks.

The healthy bottom line: Nutrient-dense munching doesn't get much better than this. Count on nabbing 12 grams of protein, 6 grams of fiber and 4.5 grams of heart-healthy fats.

8. Antipasto Plate (167 calories)
Love eating little bits of everything? Plate a few cubes of feta cheese (1 ounce), 3 small olives of any variety, 10 cherry tomatoes, 4 carrot sticks and 1 large whole grain cracker sheet (such as Ryvita Fruit 'n Nut Crunch Crispbread). Cutting back on sodium? Switch to a low-salt cheese, such as Alpine Lace Reduced Sodium Muenster or Low Sodium Boar's Head Gold Label Imported Swiss.

The healthy bottom line: The veggies are packed with bone-strengthening calcium and a little bit of lots of nutrients and disease-fighting chemicals. The olives boast heart-healthy fat.

9. Guacamole & Black Bean Chips (191 calories)
Improve your chip nutritional I.Q. with the new kid on the block: gluten-free Beanitos, black bean snack chips made with black beans and brown rice. Go for 10 chips with 3 tablespoons of homemade guacamole or a healthful store-bought variety like Wholly Guacamole Classic. Yes, avocados are high in fat, but it's a heart-healthy monounsaturated fat that helps lower cholesterol.

The healthy bottom line: With more than double the protein of corn and potato chips and a whopping 5 grams of fiber, the low-glycemic chips are great for keeping blood sugar stable.

10. Skinny Latte & 10 Almonds (150 calories)

Iced in the summer or hot in the winter, coffee is the perfect snack when you want to sip your way to smart nutrition. The antioxidant-rich brew is good for aging muscles, especially when spiked with a healthy dose of skim-milk protein and a side of heart-healthy nuts. Don't worry about the slight calorie range at different coffee shops — just go for the 16-ounce size and add skim or soy milk to make it skinny. Making latte at home? Try this recipe.

The healthy bottom line: Milk (or soy milk) nets appetite-quenching protein and bone-strengthening calcium. But the coffee's not too shabby either: New studies suggest caffeine may help strengthen older muscles.

Need more snack ideas? Check out suggestions from health organizations like the American Heart Association and the American Diabetes Association.

EATING TO CURE DIABETES TYPE 2

How changes in diet can reverse the disease — and the 3 surprising foods that really help

---

By Maureen Callahan

Maureen Callahan is a registered dietitian, recipe developer and lead author of the Health.com diet book review series.

Not so long ago a diagnosis of Type 2 diabetes at 50 or 60 seemed final, one of those no-turning-back kind of moments. Chances are the doctor told you the disease could be managed, but a return to a day when blood sugars might fall back into normal range (less than 126 mg/dl) was not on the table. An amazing new study suggests just the opposite. If you're willing to make changes in what you eat and ramp up your activity levels, diabetes could be put into full or partial remission.

How so? It can all be summed up in two words: lose weight.

In a study by the Centers for Disease Control and Prevention, researchers randomly assigned 4,500 overweight Type 2 diabetics to either an intensive diet and exercise boot camp-style intervention or a less stringent weight-loss education program.

The group given an intensive lifestyle intervention had weekly group and individual counseling sessions on what to eat and how to exercise for six months straight. (The follow-up dropped to three times a month for the next six months, then twice a month, along with periodic group refresher courses, for years two through four.)

The second group received social support, along with advice on diet and physical activity, but only three times a year and as part of a group, not individually.

Not surprisingly, the group given intensive diet and lifestyle counseling showed the most success. More important, 11.5 percent of the intensive lifestyle intervention group saw partial or complete remission of diabetes (remission was defined as blood sugars less than 126 mg/dl and hemoglobin A1c of less than 6.5 percent) at the one-year mark. Compare that figure to the other group's success rate: 2 percent.

The researchers, who published their study in December's Journal of the American Medical Association, are not the first to find that weight loss can turn diabetes around.

Maybe you're heard personal anecdotes like that of Bob Smietana, a reporter from The Tennessean. He wrote an inspiring account in USA Today of how diet and exercise made a dramatic impact on his blood sugar levels after a recent diagnosis of Type 2 diabetes.

Then there's the groundbreaking Why WAIT weight-loss program from the Harvard-affiliated Joslin Diabetes Center. It has helped 450 people with Type 2 diabetes lose an average of 24 pounds and reduce their medication and insulin amounts. In other words, it has changed the course of their diabetes. Dr. Osama Hamdy, assistant professor of medicine and a physician at Joslin, recently told the Harvard Gazette, "You can reverse the cycle if it's early enough, before there's significant damage to the pancreas." Studies show that people with diabetes or prediabetes who lose just 7 percent of their body weight can improve their body's sensitivity to insulin an astonishing 57 percent.

So how do you eat to cure diabetes and achieve this weight loss? Not with one single or magical food, according to the American

Diabetes Association. The best strategy is to eat a variety of healthy foods, including vegetables, whole grains, fruits, non-fat dairy, beans, lean meats and fish. "Make sure your choices from each food group provide the highest quality nutrients you can find," the ADA says, by picking foods "rich in vitamins, minerals and fiber over those that are processed."

And while you're cleaning up eating habits and working to lose weight, it might not hurt to add these three foods to your weight-loss formula. Preliminary findings suggest they can have a positive impact on managing blood sugar.

Vinegar Sipping water sweetened lightly with a sugar substitute and laced with 20 grams of vinegar a few minutes before meals improved insulin sensitivity in a small group of subjects who either had Type 2 diabetes or were insulin resistant, according to a 2004 study in Diabetes Care. In a video interview with WedMD, lead researcher Carol Johnston, director of the nutrition program at Arizona State University, explains why: "Both the blood glucose and insulin were better managed after the meal when they consumed vinegar. It appears the vinegar mimics the effects of both acrabose and metformin, which are two of the commonly prescribed medications for diabetics."

Coffee Over the last decade or so, multiple studies have observed a link between high intakes of coffee and decaf coffee and a reduced risk of diabetes. A 2012 Japanese study randomized volunteers into two groups for 16 weeks, letting one group drink five cups of decaf per day and another drink five cups of regular coffee. After measuring glucose and insulin concentrations in both groups, researchers suggested both types of coffee might boost glucose tolerance.

A 2011 Harvard study of coffee drinkers suggests that compounds in coffee might indirectly protect against diabetes by helping liver and fat cells function. "Often people think of coffee as just a vehicle for caffeine, but it's actually a very complex beverage with hundreds and hundreds of different compounds in it," said Rob van Dam, an assistant professor in the Department of Nutrition at Harvard. So it may take some time for researchers to tease out the helpful ingredients.

Cinnamon Researchers reporting in a 2012 issue of the International Journal of Preventive Medicine found that cinnamon supplements (3 grams per day) helped improve fasting blood glucose levels, hemoglobin A1C levels and other measures of glycemic status in a small group of Type 2 diabetics. That finding goes right along with an earlier 2009 study from the United Kingdom. "More research is needed to confirm these findings and determine how cinnamon supplementation leads to these benefits," said Dr. M. Regina Castro, an endocrinologist at the Mayo Clinic. "One theory is that cinnamon increases insulin action."

5 SIMPLE WAYS TO SLASH YOUR SALT INTAKE

You know excess sodium is bad for you, but what can you do about it? Here are some ways to start cutting back

---

By Gina Roberts-Grey

Gina Roberts-Grey is an award-wining writer who has written nearly 2,000 articles spanning a broad spectrum of health topics. Her features have appeared within numerous magazines and websites.

We all know that consuming too much salt is bad for us — but mounting scientific evidence indicates it's even worse than we thought. More people in midlife and beyond are starting to get serious about slashing their salt intake to ward off heart disease and other life-threatening conditions. But they face an uphill climb.

Adults in the United States consume an average of 3,400 mg of sodium a day, more than double the 1,500 that the American Heart Association recommends. All that excess sodium contributes to high blood pressure, heart attacks and an increased risk of stroke, osteoporosis, stomach cancer and kidney disease.

Salt can also be bad for your bones. A study presented by Japanese researchers last month at the Endocrine Society's annual meeting in San Francisco found that a diet too high in salt can increase a postmenopausal woman's risk of breaking a bone, particularly a hip, regardless of her bone density. Older women in the study with the highest concentration of sodium in their diets appeared to be at least four times more likely to suffer fractures than women with the most modest consumption. (The study took place in Japan, where the average daily sodium consumption of nearly 4,000 mg is even higher than in the U.S.)

A separate study, directed by Harvard and Yale medical school researchers and published in the journal *Nature* in March, found that excessive salt in the body may also stimulate aggressive cells that trigger autoimmune diseases like multiple sclerosis and psoriasis. The study was inspired by the observation that eating fast-food appeared to boost production of inflammatory cells that could attack healthy tissue.

In a subsequent study of mice, the research team found adding salt to the animals' diet sparked production of a type of T cell associated with autoimmune diseases. The mice eating the high-salt diet were also prone to developing a more severe type of MS than others.

If Americans were to cut their average sodium intake to 1,500 mg a day, the heart association estimates, the result would be a nearly 26 percent decrease in high blood pressure and a savings of more than $26 billion in annual health care costs.

How Can You Cut the Salt?

Salt is everywhere in our diet, especially in processed and frozen-food products. Further, nutritionists believe that a drastic cold-turkey reduction, unless mandated by a medical condition, is unlikely to succeed. Most people slide back into old habits after attempting a radical change in diet. The best approach: gradual, reasonable steps toward a new, healthier regimen. Consider starting with these five steps to reduce your salt intake.

1. **Rethink breakfast cereal** Yes, the whole grains can be a healthy choice, but many varieties still contain as much as 150 mg (or more) of sodium in a single cup.

Sodium is added to cereals, especially so-called "healthy" ones, to make them more palatable, says Amanda Gilley, a registered dietician and chef at LifeBridge Health & Fitness in Baltimore. "In fact, many products that market themselves as healthy or low-fat typically have extra sodium and sugar to help boost the taste."

As Pulitzer Prize–winning investigative reporter Michael Moss of the New York Times revealed in his book, *Salt Sugar Fat: How the Food Giants Hooked Us*, food companies often up the salt or sugar in their products when they reduce the fat, hoping consumers focused on low-fat items won't notice.

Swap cereal for oatmeal made with steel-cut oats. If you like, top it with fresh blueberries. This way, there's virtually no sodium in your bowl, making it a healthy way to start the day.

2. **Simplify boiling water** Most home cooks habitually add a dash of salt to the water they boil for pasta because it increases the boiling point and boosts flavor. But that dash can have as much as 200 mg of sodium, says Gilley, who advises skipping that step going forward.

She also suggests that you coat your dish with a homemade sauce — using a recipe that doesn't call for salt — instead of opening a sodium-laden store-bought bottle. "If time is of the essence," she says, "look for a low-sodium tomato sauce, but stay away from brands that are labeled 'reduced sodium' as these still contain a significant amount."

3. **Drop the pizza** Once and for all, we need to classify pizza as junk food and not a valid meal, says Mary Hartley, a registered dietician and nutritionist in Brooklyn, N.Y. Two slices of a 14-inch pepperoni pizza can have upwards of 1,280 mgs of salt, depending on the type and volume of sauce and topping. "A Big Mac with medium fries

has 1,310 milligrams of sodium," she says, "but many still think of pizza as being a healthier option."

Can't imagine a life without slices? That's fine, Hartley says. Just make it yourself instead of ordering in. Make your crust from a low-sodium recipe — supermarket kits are loaded with salt. Use fresh vegetables like sliced tomato, green peppers and broccoli for toppings instead of sodium-filled meats like pepperoni or sausage. To spice it up, deploy fresh basil and garlic or a dash of oregano and, of course, use low-sodium cheese.

4. Use kosher salt Substituting this larger, coarser-grained salt for fine table salt can quickly slash your sodium consumption by 20 percent because its shape and texture give it less sodium by volume. (Sea salt provides the same benefit, but only if you use a coarse-grained variety). Standard table salt delivers 590 mg of sodium per quarter-teaspoon, whereas kosher salt has 480.

"Better yet, instead of salting food during cooking," Hartley says, "just add a few grains of kosher salt to your food at the table to get a pungent burst of flavor with much less sodium."

Or skip the salt altogether and use lower-sodium flavor enhancers like black pepper and turmeric; fresh basil and dried herbs; olive oil, lemon juice, wine and vinegar; or roots such as garlic and ginger.

5. Beware the chicken We often consider turkey and chicken healthy alternatives to red meat, but we should also be aware of their potentially high sodium content, which can be traced to the saltwater solution producers typically inject into poultry during processing. "This adds flavor and weight to the meat, and it plumps up the poultry," says Steve Hoad of Emma's Family Farm in Windsor, Maine, "although we process birds without salt or water added and they still taste very good."

While boneless, skinless chicken breast not treated with saltwater typically carries 50 to 75 mg of sodium per 4-ounce serving,

Hartley says, "enhanced chicken often delivers over 400 milligrams of sodium per serving."

About a third of the fresh chicken found in supermarket cases has been synthetically saturated with saltwater, Hartley says. To spot (and avoid) the affected poultry, you've got to read the labels very carefully. Look for the phrase "Enhanced with up to 15 percent chicken broth" within the package's fine print, she advises, and be aware that poultry enhanced with saltwater can still be called "all natural" if the ingredients in the solution meet the U.S. Department of Agriculture's definition of "natural."

THE 3 BEST WAYS TO EAT FOR A HEALTHY HEART

It's not so much the specific foods, but your overall eating pattern. Which plan is right for you?

By Maureen Callahan

Maureen Callahan is a registered dietitian, recipe developer and lead author of the Health.com diet book review series.

Multiple factors influence the development and progression of cardiovascular disease. So while most experts agree that diet plays a big role in prevention and treatment of heart disease, there are definite controversies surrounding which diet is best. Still, general agreement is that a diet for heart health focuses on an overall eating pattern rather than particular foods that can lower cholesterol levels, blood pressure or heart disease risk.

As far as overall patterns go, the Mediterranean Diet still holds top honors in many health organizations. Yet two newer regimens are coming to light that might protect the heart just as well, if not better.

Which plan is best for you? Here's a look at the latest findings and a brief description of each.

The Mediterranean Diet

The specifics Billed as the traditional diet of sun-drenched Mediterranean locales, this plan is loosely defined as one that focuses on filling the plate with plenty of fruits, vegetables, whole grains and moderate amounts of healthy fats, like nuts and olive oil. Fish and poultry, eaten in moderate amounts, are preferred over red and processed meats. Dairy products and sweets are kept to a minimum, but a little wine with meals is fine.

The science Multiple studies have linked a Mediterranean eating style with lower heart disease risk. Yet, a 2013 clinical study published in the New England Journal of Medicine gives such strong support to the diet's positive impact that researchers ended up stopping the study early, after almost five years, because the results were so clear it would have been unethical to continue.

University of Barcelona scientists divided nearly 7,500 volunteers age 55 to 80 into three groups and followed them for five years. One group consumed a low-fat diet; the two others ate a Mediterranean-style diet enhanced with either nuts or olive oil. Participants following either Mediterranean plan lowered cardiovascular disease endpoints — heart attacks, stroke, death — a whopping 30 percent. Current thinking is that this style diet could be even as effective as drug therapy but without negative drug side effects.

"Even the best available drugs, like statins, reduce heart disease by about 25 percent, which is in the same ballpark as the Mediterranean diet," Walter Willett, chair of the Department of Nutrition at Harvard School of Public Health, said in the Boston Globe. "But the statins increase the risk of diabetes, whereas this diet can help reduce the risk."

Is it for you? Probably. It's an easy plan to follow since the emphasis isn't on restricting fat but rather on eating moderate amounts of healthy fats like nuts, olive oil and avocados. A splash or two of red wine isn't hard to swallow either. Check out the Mayo Clinic for recipes and more details.

The Anti-Inflammatory Diet

The specifics The theory is that chronic or low-grade levels of inflammation (the same body response that helps you heal from a wound, but on a much milder level) are bad for the heart and health in general. Dr. Stephen Sinatra, an integrative cardiologist, goes so far as to suggest that inflammation, not elevated cholesterol levels, is the real cause of heart disease.

Whether it is or not, anti-inflammatory diets are a mixed bag of advice depending on which website or book you read. Foods to avoid could include everything from omega 6 fatty acids found in vegetable oils, sugar and processed foods to common allergens, like soy, peanuts and wheat.

The science One word describes the scientific back-up for anti-inflammation eating plans: shaky. The consensus is there's a lot more research to be done about inflammation — and the foods that might tame it — before any real diet-heart disease links can be confirmed.

Researchers at the Helfgott Research Institute and the General Clinical Research Center at Oregon Health and Science University hope to tackle the anti-inflammatory diet/disease link with a group of diabetics and pre-diabetics. They want study participants to follow the anti-inflammatory diet or one based on American Diabetic Association recommendations for six weeks. "If the anti-inflammatory diet reduces inflammatory cytokines," they say, "it may be an important diet for people with various conditions, including inflammatory autoimmune diseases, such as multiple sclerosis, rheumatoid arthritis and IDDM," or type I diabetes.

As for the connection between heart disease and inflammation, "My best advice is to stay tuned," says Dr. Brent Bauer of the Mayo Clinic. "This is a huge area of interest in the medical world and there are bound to be discoveries down the road that can improve well-being and the quality of health."

Is it for you? Maybe. Most anti-inflammatory diets promote good choices that are remarkably similar to a Mediterranean-style way of eating. But the foods they restrict — for example, wheat (gluten), dairy and nightshade vegetables (peppers, eggplant, tomatoes and potatoes) — might be unnecessary changes for most people.

The Plant-Based Diet

The specifics The all-plant diet that President Bill Clinton endorses is actually code for a vegan diet that eschews all animal products and also limits fat, including such heart-healthy ones as olive oil, avocados and nuts.

The science There are no randomized, double-blind, controlled clinical trials that have tested the vegan diet and its relationship to cardiovascular events, like heart attack or stroke. But even as far back as 1998, an editorial in the Journal of the American College of Nutrition suggested that several international studies have linked plant-based diets to a lower risk for ischemic heart disease. And retired Cleveland Clinic cardiologist Dr. Caldwell B. Esselstyn Jr., a cardiologist who worked at the Cleveland Clinic, offers 20 years of evidence from his patients showing dramatic drops in cholesterol and a widening of coronary arteries (based on angiograms) and what he calls a reversal of heart disease with a vegan, low oil diet. "In the world's poorer nations, many people subsist on a primarily plant-based diet, which is far healthier, especially in terms of heart disease," Esselstyn said in the journal Preventive Cardiology.

Is it for you? It's not going to be popular with meat lovers or those who don't want to limit healthy fats, like olive oil. And it's far, far, different from the high-fat, highly processed Western diet. But groaning and complaining aside, this diet is entirely doable, particularly if you love, or at least keep an open mind about, meals that highlight fresh fruits, vegetables, legumes and whole grains.

ABOUT NEXT AVENUE

America is in the midst of an age boom and with it, an amazing transition. In general, those of us over the age of 50 are expected to live longer than any previous generation.

We're in the process of creating a new life stage that lies somewhere between young adulthood and "old-old" adulthood. This stage doesn't have a name. We call it Adult Part 2. And if you're reading this you're probably smack dab in it.

You're aware that many years of life lie ahead of you and, very likely, you have a different set of expectations for these "bonus years" than you had for earlier adulthood. You sense that you can somehow apply your knowledge and experiences in a meaningful way. Yet you may not know exactly how to achieve this new vision or see all the many possibilities available to you as you navigate the physical, health, work, and financial shifts that inevitably accompany this phase.

Enter **Next Avenue**. We're a group of public television people and journalists who, for the most part, are experiencing the very same things you are. Like you, we see both challenges and opportunities and we recognize that what we could all use right about now is an abundance of reliable information that can help us figure out what's, well, next.

So we aim to deliver that—in a way that's both smart and accessible.

Thanks for walking with us down Next Avenue.

ABOUT DONNA SAPOLIN

As Founding Editor of Next Avenue, Donna Sapolin has been steeped in the issues and stories of Adult, Part 2. A longtime magazine editor and writer, she curated this collection from writings that originally appeared on nextavenue.org.

For more Next Avenue e-books, please visit the PBS Digital Shop!

Made in the USA
Monee, IL
04 November 2026

67374661R00036